Keto Chaffle

Recipes

For Beginners 2021

40 Quick And Easy Recipes For Weight Loss And Boost Brain Health.

Dorothy F.Brown

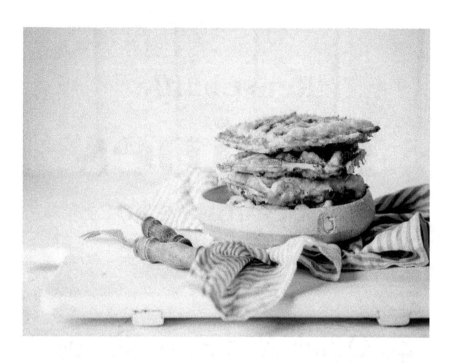

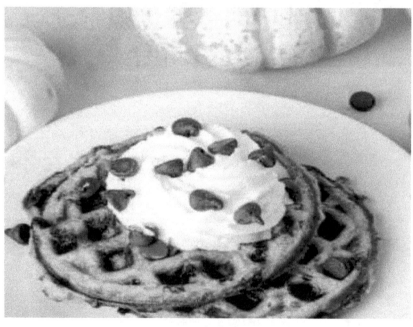

Table of Contents

extends to creating a secondary or tertiary copy of the work or a recorded copy and is only allowed with the express written consent from the Publisher. All additional right reserved.

The information in the following pages is broadly considered a truthful and accurate account of facts and as such, any inattention, use, or misuse of the information in question by the reader will render any resulting actions solely under their purview. There are no scenarios in which the publisher or the original author of this work can be in any fashion deemed liable for any hardship or damages that may befall them after undertaking information described herein.

Additionally, the information in the following pages is intended only for informational purposes and should thus be thought of as universal. As befitting its nature, it is presented without assurance regarding its prolonged validity or interim quality. Trademarks that are mentioned are done without written consent and can in no way be considered an endorsement from the trademark holder.

INTRODUCTION

K eto Diet is a high-fat, low-carb diet that is an increasingly popular way to lose weight. Keto is short for "ketosis", which occurs when the body has depleted its sugar stores, so it burns stored fat instead of glucose in order to produce energy.

Losing weight on a keto diet sounds pretty easy; just eat a few bacon sandwiches and you'll be slimmer in no time. However, there are drawbacks to this diet, including very low levels of vegetables and fruit (so important for fiber and other nutrients) as well as constipation from lack of dietary fiber. Here are some tips:

- It's important to drink plenty of water, not only because you may be eating more sodium than you need, but because staying hydrated will help your body process proteins and fats more efficiently.

- For best results, stay away from most fruits and vegetables. Some berries are allowed; others aren't.

Vegetables that are considered "low in carbs" or "leafy greens" are fine—but there is a difference between low-carb and high-fiber. As a rule of thumb, if it looks like it has the texture of tree bark or is covered with seeds or bulbs (e.g., artichokes), it probably has a lot of carbs and should be avoided.

- Be careful with spices, which tend to have a lot of sugar; salt is OK. It can be easy to go overboard on spices.

- Eat plenty of salmon, tuna and egg whites. Meat—including beef, chicken, pork and lamb—should comprise 20 to 25 percent of your total diet. (Be aware that "lean" meat is often not very lean. Be prepared to trim off most of that fat before cooking.) A little bacon or sausage is fine, too.

- Avoid condiments and sauces, including barbecue sauce and ketchup. These are full of sugar and other unhealthy ingredients.

- Drink mostly water (or unsweetened drinks such as tea or coffee). Try to avoid drinks with a lot of added sugar, like fruit juice or alcohol. If you choose to drink wine, go for the dry stuff—red wine is best.

Now, for Chaffles.

What is Chaffle?

Keto chaffle recipe is a versatile and easy-to-make low carb pancake that only requires 2 ingredients. It's a way to satisfy your sweet cravings while staying keto!

Chaffle is made from cheese and eggs. You will need grated cheddar cheese (use any kind of cheese you have on hand) and eggs, beaten together, then fried in a pan with butter or coconut oil.

Chaffles are perfect for a low carb breakfast, lunch or dinner and can be a treat right out of the pan, with butter!

Why Keto and Chaffle is a perfect combination?

Keto Chaffle is a great way to satisfy your sweet cravings while staying 100% in ketosis. It helps you feel fuller for longer but at the same time it's not a high carb treat.

Chaffle gives you a lot of energy and it's an easy way to prepare breakfast if you want it to be ready quickly when you get up or even if you're in a hurry so it can be prepared on the go without any issues.

Keto Chaffle tastes amazing plain, with butter or with any toppings you like and it can also be used as sandwich bread substitute.

KETOGENIC DIET AND ITS BENEFITS

What is Ketogenic Diet?

The ketogenic diet is a low-carb, high-fat diet. This means that the macronutrient ratio of your diet should consist mainly of fat and protein with only a small percentage of carbohydrates.

The idea behind the ketogenic diet is to force your body to use fat rather than glucose as its primary fuel source. When we are in ketosis, we can function on almost any fuel source.

Benefits of the Ketogenic Diet

The benefits of the ketogenic diet are as follows:

1. No need to count calories.

On this diet, you can eat as much as you want. Since there are no grains, the carbohydrates in the diet are very low, and so you will not take in many calories.

2. There is no need to spend a lot of money on expensive foods.

Since this diet is high in fat, one of the cheapest sources of fat is chicken thighs and legs and other skinless poultry parts or meats from around the animal, such as organ meats (heart, liver, etc.).

3. Low levels of Beta-hydroxybutyrate (ketone body) is suitable for brain health

The ketogenic diet can increase the level of ketone bodies by 10 times than normal dietary levels through fat metabolism.

4. Decreased risk of heart disease

Many people can lower their LDL (bad) cholesterol by 75-90% and triglyceride levels by 60%.

5. Less inflammation

Because there are no carbohydrates in the ketogenic diet, your body becomes very efficient at burning ketones as fuel. This is excellent news if you have an autoimmune disorder like rheumatoid arthritis or Crohn's disease because inflammation is often linked to autoimmune problems.

6. Fast weight loss

People usually start losing weight within two weeks of starting the diet.

7. Increased energy levels

The ketogenic diet can increase your energy levels because you will be consuming a high-fat diet with very few carbohydrates.

8. No constant hunger

When people are on a ketogenic diet, they are in "ketosis." This means that their bodies are using fat as an almost complete fuel source. This is the opposite of how most people function in a non-ketogenic state, which usually involves using carbohydrates (sugars) as a practically whole fuel source. Because the ketogenic diet is so different, the body is forced to use fat as its primary fuel source to function. This means you won't be hungry all the time once you get the hang of it.

9. No need for cheat meals

Since carbohydrates are reduced in this diet, cheating on the ketogenic diet will not help you lose weight because your body does not have carbohydrates stored to keep your metabolism running, being that fat is used instead of sugar/carbs.

10. No need to buy expensive supplements

Since the diet is not very restrictive, you won't need to buy many supplements besides vitamin D3 if you are deficient.

11. You can gain muscle and lose fat at the same time

When you do strength training with a ketogenic diet, the weight loss is due to body fat (adipose tissue), not muscle mass. Many people find it difficult to lose weight because they are losing muscle mass and body fat, which is not suitable for overall health. However, because this diet encourages protein consumption at every meal, as well as healthy fats, your amino acid intake will be sufficient to preserve your muscles without inhibiting your weight loss.

Foods Allowed

Here is the list of foods you can eat during the ketogenic diet:

1. Meat, poultry, fish, shellfish, and eggs from pasture-fed animals (animals are fed a grass-fed diet)

2. Fish and seafood caught in the wild

3. Eggs from pastured hens

4. Vegetables, including root vegetables such as beets and carrots and leafy greens such as spinach and kale.

5. Healthy fats such as coconut oil or olive oil that can be used in place of butter or other oils (11 grams per day maximum)

6. Nuts and seeds such as macadamia nuts, walnuts, and pumpkin seeds

7. Low to moderate amounts of dairy products such as yogurt and cheese

8. Non-starchy vegetables such as broccoli, cauliflower, and other cruciferous vegetables

9. Fruits

Foods That Are Not Allowed

Foods that are not allowed

When following the keto diet, you will want to avoid eating the following foods:

1. Grains including wheat, oats, rice, and corn
2. Sugar, including honey, maple syrup, and sugar in all its forms
3. Vegetable oils such as canola, sunflower, and soybean oil
4. Trans fats such as margarine and vegetable shortening
5. Juices and sugary drinks such as soda, fruit juices with added sugar or artificial sweeteners, or milk alternatives made with grains such as almond milk
6. Grain-based dairy products such as butter and yogurt
7. Legumes such as beans, soybeans, and peanuts
8. Starchy vegetables such as potatoes, peas, and corn
9. Processed foods of any kind, including sauces and any food that contains a high percentage of preservatives
10. Beer (pure alcohol)

11. Low-fat or nonfat dairy products such as yogurt and cheese (dairy products that are low in fat but have carbohydrates)

12. Fruit juices with added sugars or artificial sweeteners

Volume (liquid)

US Customary	Metric
1/8 teaspoon	.6 ml
1/4 teaspoon	1.2 ml
1/2 teaspoon	2.5 ml
3/4 teaspoon	3.7 ml
1 teaspoon	5 ml
1 tablespoon	15 ml
2 tablespoon or 1 fluid ounce	30 ml
1/4 cup or 2 fluid ounces	59 ml
1/3 cup	79 ml
1/2 cup	118 ml
2/3 cup	158 ml
3/4 cup	177 ml
1 cup or 8 fluid ounces	237 ml
2 cups or 1 pint	473 ml
4 cups or 1 quart	946 ml
8 cups or 1/2 gallon	1.9 liters
1 gallon	3.8 liters

Weight (mass)

US contemporary (ounces)	Metric (grams)
1/2 ounce	14 grams
1 ounce	28 grams
3 ounces	85 grams
3.53 ounces	100 grams
4 ounces	113 grams
8 ounces	227 grams
12 ounces	340 grams
16 ounces or 1 pound	454 grams

Volume Equivalents (liquid)*

3 teaspoons	1 tablespoon	0.5 fluid ounce
2 tablespoons	1/8 cup	1 fluid ounce
4 tablespoons	1/4 cup	2 fluid ounces
5 1/3 tablespoons	1/3 cup	2.7 fluid ounces
8 tablespoons	1/2 cup	4 fluid ounces
12 tablespoons	3/4 cup	6 fluid ounces
16 tablespoons	1 cup	8 fluid ounces
2 cups	1 pint	16 fluid ounces

BREAKFAST CHAFFLE RECIPES

1. Morning Chaffles With Berries

Preparation Time: 10 minutes

Cooking Time: 5 Minutes

Servings: 4

Ingredients:

- 1 cup egg whites
- 1 cup cheddar cheese, shredded
- ¼ cup almond flour
- ¼ cup heavy cream
- TOPPING
- 4 oz. raspberries
- 4 oz. strawberries.
- 1 oz. keto chocolate flakes
- 1 oz. feta cheese.

Directions:

1. Preheat your square waffle maker and grease with cooking spray.
2. Beat egg white in a small bowl with flour.
3. Add shredded cheese to the egg whites and flour mixture and mix well.
4. Add cream and cheese to the egg mixture.
5. Pour Chaffles batter in a waffle maker and close the lid.

6. Cook chaffles for about 4 minutes Utes until crispy and brown.
7. Carefully remove chaffles from the maker.
8. Serve with berries, cheese, and chocolate on top.
9. Enjoy!

Nutrition:

- Protein: 28% 68 kcal
- Fat: 67% 163 kcal
- Carbohydrates: 5% 12 kcal

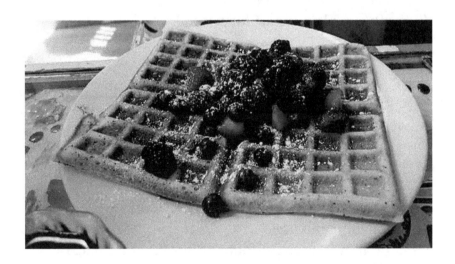

2. Mixed Berry & Vanilla Chaffles

Preparation time: 10 minutes

Cooking time: 28 minutes

Servings: 4

Ingredients:

- 1 egg, beaten
- ½ cup finely grated mozzarella cheese
- 1 tbsp cream cheese, softened
- 1 tbsp sugar-free maple syrup
- 2 strawberries, sliced
- 2 raspberries, slices
- ¼ tsp blackberry extract
- ¼ tsp vanilla extract
- ½ cup plain yogurt for serving

Directions:

1. Preheat the waffle iron.
2. In a medium bowl, mix all the ingredients except the yogurt.
3. Open the iron, lightly grease with cooking spray and pour in a quarter of the mixture.
4. Close the iron and cook until golden brown and crispy, 7 minutes.
5. Remove the chaffle onto a plate and set aside.
6. Make three more chaffles with the remaining mixture.
7. To serve: top with the yogurt and enjoy.

Nutrition:

- Calories: 99 Cal
- Total Fat: 8 g
- Saturated Fat: 0 g
- Cholesterol: 0 mg
- Sodium: 0 mg
- Total Carbs: 4 g

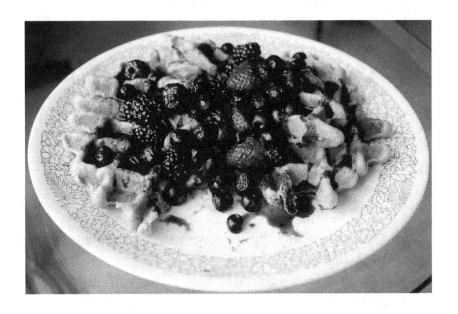

3. Ham and Cheddar Chaffles

Preparation time: 15 minutes

Cooking time: 28 minutes

Servings: 4

Ingredients:

- 1 cup finely shredded parsnips, steamed
- 8 oz ham, diced
- 2 eggs, beaten
- 1 ½ cups finely grated cheddar cheese
- ½ tsp garlic powder
- 2 tbsp chopped fresh parsley leaves
- ¼ tsp smoked paprika
- ½ tsp dried thyme
- Salt and freshly ground black pepper to taste

Directions:

1. Preheat the waffle iron.
2. In a medium bowl, mix all the ingredients.
3. Open the iron, lightly grease with cooking spray and pour in a quarter of the mixture.
4. Close the iron and cook until crispy, 7 minutes.
5. Remove the chaffle onto a plate and set aside.
6. Make three more chaffles using the remaining mixture.
7. Serve afterward.

Nutrition:

- Calories: 126 Cal
- Total Fat: 15 g
- Saturated Fat: 4 g
- Cholesterol: 26 mg
- Sodium: 41 mg
- Total Carbs: 13 g

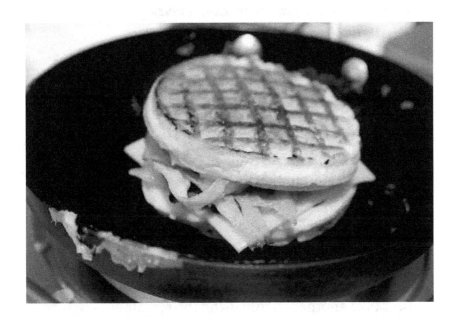

4. Savory Gruyere and Chives Chaffles

Preparation time: 15 minutes

Cooking time: 14 minutes

Servings: 2

Ingredients:

- 2 eggs, beaten
- 1 cup finely grated Gruyere cheese
- 2 tbsp finely grated cheddar cheese
- 1/8 tsp freshly ground black pepper
- 3 tbsp minced fresh chives + more for garnishing
- 2 sunshine fried eggs for topping

Directions:

1. Preheat the waffle iron.
2. In a medium bowl, mix the eggs, cheeses, black pepper, and chives.
3. Open the iron and pour in half of the mixture.
4. Close the iron and cook until brown and crispy, 7 minutes.
5. Remove the chaffle onto a plate and set aside.
6. Make another chaffle using the remaining mixture.
7. Top each chaffle with one fried egg each, garnish with the chives and serve.

Nutrition:

- Calories: 87 Cal
- Total Fat: 6 g
- Saturated Fat: 4 g
- Cholesterol: 34 mg
- Sodium: 46 mg
- Total Carbs: 5 g

5. Chicken Quesadilla Chaffle

Preparation time: 10 minutes

Cooking time: 14 minutes

Servings: 2

Ingredients:

- 1 egg, beaten
- ¼ tsp taco seasoning
- 1/3 cup finely grated cheddar cheese
- 1/3 cup cooked chopped chicken

Directions:

1. Preheat the waffle iron.
2. In a medium bowl, mix the eggs, taco seasoning, and cheddar cheese. Add the chicken and combine well.
3. Open the iron, lightly grease with cooking spray and pour in half of the mixture.
4. Close the iron and cook until brown and crispy, 7 minutes.
5. Remove the chaffle onto a plate and set aside.
6. Make another chaffle using the remaining mixture.
7. Serve afterward.

Nutrition:

Calories: 146 Cal

Total Fat: 17 g

Saturated Fat: 12 g

Cholesterol: 56 mg

Sodium: 79 mg

Total Carbs: 12 g

6. Bacon-Cheddar Biscuit Chaffle

Preparation time: 10 minutes

Cooking time: 28 minutes

Servings: 4

Ingredients:

- 1 egg, beaten
- 2 tbsp. almond flour
- 2 tbsp. ground flaxseed
- 3 bacon slices, cooked and chopped
- ¼ cup heavy cream
- 1 ½ tbsp. melted butter
- ½ cup finely grated Gruyere cheese
- ½ cup finely grated cheddar cheese
- ¼ tsp. erythritol
- ½ tsp. onion powder
- ½ tsp. garlic salt
- ½ tbsp. dried parsley
- ½ tbsp. baking powder
- ¼ tsp. baking soda

Directions:

1. Preheat the waffle iron.
2. Meanwhile, in a medium bowl, whisk all the ingredients until smooth batter forms.
3. Open the iron, pour a quarter of the mixture into the iron, close and cooking until crispy, 6 to 7 minutes.
4. Remove the chaffle onto a plate and set aside.
5. Make three more Chaffles with the remaining batter.
6. Allow cooling and serve afterward.

Nutrition:

- Calories: 207 kcal
- Protein: 22.68 g
- Fat: 11.89 g
- Carbohydrates: 1.17 g

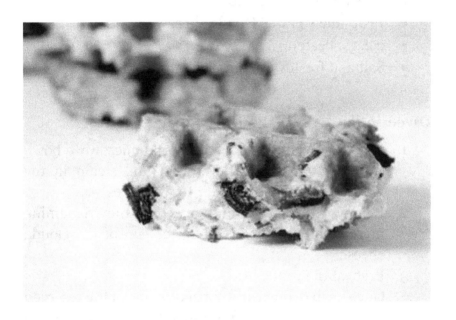

7. Turnip Hash Brown Chaffles

Preparation time: 10 minutes

Cooking time: 42 minutes

Servings: 6

Ingredients:

- 1 large turnip, peeled and shredded
- ½ medium white onion, minced
- 2 garlic cloves, pressed
- 1 cup finely grated Gouda cheese
- 2 eggs, beaten
- Salt and freshly ground black pepper to taste

Directions:

1. Pour the turnips in a medium safe microwave bowl, sprinkle with 1 tbsp. of water, and steam in the microwave until softened, 1 to 2 minutes.
2. Remove the bowl and mix in the remaining ingredients except for a quarter cup of the Gouda cheese.
3. Preheat the waffle iron.
4. Once heated, open and sprinkle some of the reserved cheese in the iron and top with 3 tablespoons of the mixture. Close the waffle iron and cooking until crispy, 5 minutes.
5. Open the lid, flip the chaffle and cooking further for 2 more minutes.
6. Remove the chaffle onto a plate and set aside.
7. Make five more chaffles with the remaining batter in the same proportion.
8. Allow cooling and serve afterward.

Nutrition:

- Calories: 580
- Fat: 50 g
- Net Carbohydrates: 2 g
- Protein: 30 g

8. Everything Bagel Chaffles

Preparation time: 10 minutes

Cooking time: 28 minutes

Servings: 4

Ingredients:

- 1 egg, beaten
- ½ cup finely grated Parmesan cheese
- 1 tsp. Everything Bagel seasoning
- Directions:
- Preheat the waffle iron.
- In a medium bowl, mix all the ingredients.
- Open the iron, pour in a quarter of the mixture, close, and cooking until crispy, 6 to 7 minutes.
- Remove the chaffle onto a plate and set aside.
- Make three more chaffles, allow cooling, and enjoy after.

Direction:

1. In a small bowl, whip the egg till fluffy.
2. Add 1/2 cup sharp cheddar shredded cheese to the egg mixture and mix until it's fully combined.
3. Preheat the mini Dash waffle maker.
4. Once the mini waffle iron has been heated start making the chaffles.
5. For Crispy chaffles: add 1 tsp on shredded cheese to the hot waffle iron for 30 seconds before adding the egg batter mixture.
6. Pour half the mixture into the waffle iron.
7. Sprinkle the top of the mixture with the Everything Bagel Seasoning and close the lid.

8. Cook it for about 3 to 4 minutes or until the steam stops coming up from the waffle iron. Don't open the waffle iron before 3 minutes or else you will have a melted cheese gooey mess. The cheese needs to cook long enough to form a nice crust.

Nutrition:

- Calories: 210
- Fat: 9.3g
- Net Carbs: 1.3g
- Protein: 28.9g

BASIC CHAFFLE RECIPES

9. Keto Chocolate Twinkie Copycat Chaffle

Preparation time: 5 minutes

Cooking time: 12 minutes

Servings: 3

Ingredients

- 2 tablespoons of butter (cooled)
- 2 oz. cream cheese softened
- Two large egg room temperature
- 1 teaspoon of vanilla essence
- 1/4 cup Lacanto confectionery
- Pinch of pink salt
- 1/4 cup almond flour
- 2 tablespoons coconut powder
- 2 tablespoons cocoa powder
- 1 teaspoon baking powder

Directions:

1. Preheat the Maker of Corndog.
2. Melt the butter for a minute and let it cool.
3. In the butter, whisk the eggs until smooth.
4. Remove sugar, cinnamon, sweetener and blend well.
5. Add flour of almond, flour of coconut, powder of cacao and baking powder.
6. Blend until well embedded.
7. Fill each well with ~2 tablespoons of batter and spread evenly.

8. Close the lid and let it cooking for 4 minutes.
9. Lift from the rack and cool it down.

Nutrition:

- Calories: 202
- Fat: 6.6 g
- Fiber: 5.4 g
- Carbs: 2.9 g
- Protein: 9.2 g

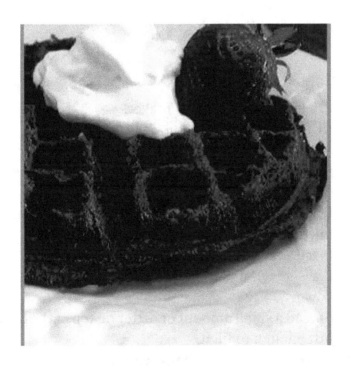

10.   Easy Corndog Chaffle Recipe

Preparation time: 10 minutes

Cooking time: 4 minutes

Servings: 5

Ingredients:

- 2 eggs
- 1 cup Mexican cheese blend
- 1 tbs almond flour
- 1/2 tsp. cornbread extract
- 1/4 tsp. salt
- hot dogs with hot dog sticks

Directions:

1. Preheat corndog waffle maker.
2. In a small bowl, whip the eggs.
3. Add the remaining ingredients except the hotdogs
4. Spray the corndog waffle maker with non-stick cooking spray.
5. Fill the corndog waffle maker with the batter halfway filled.
6. Place a stick in the hot dog.
7. Place the hot dog in the batter and slightly press down.
8. Spread a small amount of better on top of the hot dog, just enough to fill it.
9. Makes about 4 to 5 chaffle corndogs
10. Cooking the corndog chaffles for about 4 minutes or until golden brown.
11. When done, they will easily remove from the corndog waffle maker with a pair of tongs.

12. Serve with mustard, mayo, or sugar-free ketchup!

Nutrition:

- Calories: 304
- Fat: 8.3 g
- Fiber: 4.5 g
- Carbs: 1.6 g
- Protein: 7 g

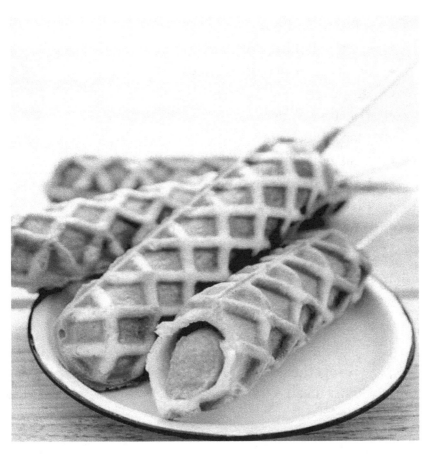

11. Krispy Kreme Copycat of Glazed Raspberry Jelly-Filled Donut

Preparation time: 10 minutes

Cooking time: 3 minutes

Servings: 4

Ingredients:

- 1 egg
- 1/4 cup Mozzarella cheese shredded
- 2 T cream cheese softened
- 1 T sweetener
- 1 T almond flour
- 1/2 tsp. Baking Powder
- 20 drops glazed donut flavoring
- Raspberry Jelly Filling Ingredients:
- 1/4 cup raspberries
- 1 tsp. chia seeds
- 1 tsp. confectioners' sweetener
- Donut Glaze Ingredients
- 1 tsp. powdered sweetener
- A few drops of water or heavy whipping cream

Directions:

1. Mix everything together to make the chaffles first.
2. Cooking for about 2 1/2-3 minutes.
3. Make the Raspberry Jelly Filling:
4. Mix together in a small pot on medium heat.
5. Gently mash raspberries.
6. Let cool.
7. Add between the layers of Chaffles.

8. Make the Donut Glaze:
9. Stir together in a small dish.
10. Drizzle on top Chaffle.

Nutrition:

- Calories: 186
- Fat: 12.1 g
- Fiber: 4.6 g
- Carbs: 11.2 g
- Protein: 7.5 g

12. Rice Krispy Treat Chaffle Copycat Recipe

Preparation time: 15 minutes

Cooking time: 5 minutes

Servings: 2

Ingredients:

Chaffle batter:

- 1 Large Egg room temp
- 2 oz. Cream Cheese softened
- 1/4 tsp. Pure Vanilla Extract
- 2 tbs Lakanto Confectioners Sweetener
- 1 oz. Pork Rinds crushed
- 1 tsp. Baking Powder
- Marshmallow Frosting:
- 1/4 c. Heavy Whipping Cream
- 1/4 tsp. Pure Vanilla Extract
- 1 tbs Lakanto Confectioners Sweetener
- 1/2 tsp. Xanthan Gum

Directions:

1. Plug in the mini waffle maker to preheat.
2. In a medium mixing bowl- Add egg, cream cheese, and vanilla.
3. Whisk until blended well.
4. Add sweetener, crushed pork rinds, and baking powder.
5. Mix until well incorporated.
6. Sprinkle extra crushed pork rinds onto waffle maker (optional).

7. Then add about 1/4 scoop of batter over, sprinkle a bit more pork rinds.
8. Cooking 3-4 minutes, then remove and cool on a wire rack.
9. Repeat for remaining batter.
10. Make the Marshmallow Frosting:
11. Whip the HWC, vanilla, and confectioners until thick and fluffy.
12. Slowly sprinkle over the xanthan gum and fold until well incorporated.
13. Spread frosting over chaffles and cut as desired, then refrigerate until set.
14. Enjoy cold or warm slightly in the microwave for 10 seconds.

Nutrition:

- Calories: 203
- Fat: 12.3 g
- Fiber: 3.1 g
- Carbs: 5.9 g
- Protein: 4.7 g

13. <u>Biscuits & Gravy Chaffle Recipe</u>

Preparation time: 10 minutes

Cooking time: 5 minutes

Servings Ingredients:

- : 4
- 2 tbs Unsalted Butter melted
- 2 Large Eggs
- 1 c. Mozzarella cheese shredded
- 1 tbs Garlic minced
- drops Cornbread Extract optional
- 1/2 tbs Lakanto Confectioners optional
- 1 tbs Almond Flour
- 1/4 tsp. Granulated Onion
- 1/4 tsp. Granulated Garlic
- 1 tsp. Dried Parsley
- 1 tsp. Baking Powder
- 1 batch Keto Sausage Biscuits and Gravy Recipe

Directions:

1. Preheat Mini Waffle Maker.
2. Melt the butter, let cool.
3. Whisk in the eggs, then fold in the shredded cheese.
4. Add the rest of ingredients and mix thoroughly.
5. Scoop 1/4 of batter onto waffle maker and cooking 4 minutes.
6. Remove and let cool on wire rack.
7. Repeat for the remaining 3 chaffles.

Nutrition:

- Calories: 270
- Fat: 10.1 g
- Fiber: 4.7 g
- Carbs: 6.3 g
- Protein: 5.8 g

14. <u>Keto Tuna Melt Chaffle Recipe</u>

Preparation time: 15 minutes

Cooking time: 8 minutes

Servings: 2

Ingredients:

- 1 packet Tuna 2.6 oz. with no water
- 1/2 cup Mozzarella cheese
- 1 egg
- pinch salt

Directions:

1. Preheat the mini waffle maker
2. In a small bowl, add the egg and whip it up.
3. Add the tuna, cheese, and salt and mix well.
4. Optional step for an extra crispy crust: Add a teaspoon of cheese to the mini waffle maker for about 30 seconds before adding the recipe mixture. This will allow the cheese to get crispy when the tuna chaffle is done cooking. I prefer this method!
5. Add 1/2 the mixture to the waffle maker and cooking it for a minimum of 4 minutes.
6. Remove it and cooking the last tuna chaffle for another 4 minutes.

Nutrition:

- Calories: 283
- Fat: 20.2 g
- Fiber: 3.3 g
- Carbs: 1.4 g
- Protein: 14.5 g

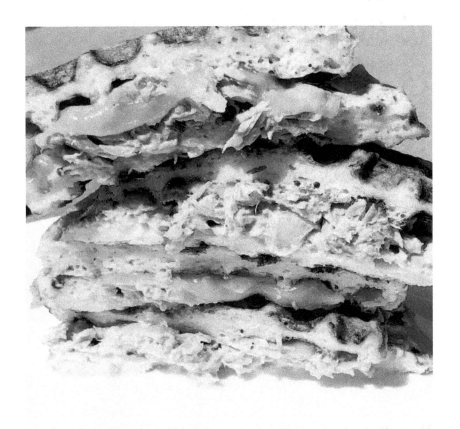

15. Blueberry & Brie Grilled Cheese Chaffle

Preparation time: 10 minutes
Cooking time: 10 minutes
Ingredients:

- 2 chaffles
- 1 t blueberry compote
- 1 oz. Wisconsin brie sliced thin
- 1 t Kerry gold butter
- Chaffle Ingredients:
- 1 egg, beaten
- 1/4 cup Mozzarella shredded
- 1 tsp. Swerve confectioners
- 1 T cream cheese softened
- 1/4 tsp. baking powder
- 1/2 tsp. vanilla extract
- Blueberry Compote Ingredients:
- 1 cup blueberries washed
- Zest of 1/2 lemon
- 1 T lemon juice freshly squeezed
- 1 T Swerve Confectioners
- 1/8 tsp. xanthan gum
- 2 T water

Directions:

1. Mix everything together.
2. Cooking 1/2 batter for 2 1/2- 3 minutes in the mini waffle maker
3. Repeat.

4. Let cool slightly on a cooling rack.
5. Blueberry Compote Directions:
6. Add everything except xanthan gum to a small saucepan. Bring to a boil, reduce heat and simmer for 5-10 minutes until it starts to thicken. Sprinkle with xanthan gum and stir well.
7. Remove from heat and let cool. Store in refrigerator until ready to use.
8. Grilled Cheese Directions:
9. Heat butter in a small pan over medium heat. Place Brie slices on a Chaffle and top with generous 1 T scoop of prepared blueberry compote.
10. Place sandwich in pan and grill, flipping once until waffle is golden and cheese has melted, about 2 minutes per side.

Nutrition:

- Calories: 273
- Fat: 16.7 g
- Fiber: 1.5 g
- Carbs: 4.1 g
- Protein: 11.8 g

16. BBQ Chicken Chaffles

Preparation time: 3 minutes

Cooking time: 8 minutes

Servings: 2

Ingredients:

- 1/3 cup cooked chicken diced
- 1/2 cup shredded cheddar cheese
- 1 tbsp. sugar-free BBQ sauce
- 1 egg
- 1 tbsp. almond flour

Directions:

1. Heat up your Dash mini waffle maker.
2. In a small bowl, mix the egg, almond flour, BBQ sauce, diced chicken, and Cheddar Cheese.
3. Add 1/2 of the batter into your mini waffle maker and cooking for 4 minutes. If they are still a bit uncooked, leave it cooking for another 2 minutes. Then cooking the rest of the batter to make a second chaffle.
4. Do not open the waffle maker before the 4-minute mark.
5. Enjoy alone or dip in BBQ Sauce or ranch dressing!

Nutrition:

- Calories: 301
- Fat: 9.7 g
- Fiber: 2.7 g
- Carbs: 5.4 g
- Protein: 15.8 g

SANDWICH AND CAKE CHAFFLE RECIPES

17. Salmon & Cream Sandwich Chaffles

Preparation time: 6 minutes

Cooking Time: 8 Minutes

Servings: 2

Ingredients:

- Chaffles
- 1 organic egg, beaten
- ½ cup cheddar cheese, shredded
- 1 tablespoon almond flour
- 1 tablespoon fresh rosemary, chopped
- Filling
- ¼ cup smoked salmon
- 1 teaspoon fresh dill, chopped
- 2 tablespoons cream

Directions:

- Preheat a mini waffle iron and then grease it.
- For chaffles: In a medium bowl, put all ingredients and with a fork, mix until well combined. Place half of the mixture into preheated waffle iron and cook for about 3–4 minutes.
- Repeat with the remaining mixture.
- Serve each chaffle with filling ingredients.

Nutrition:

- Calories: 209
- Fat: 17 g
- Protein: 6 g
- Sugar: 0.5 g

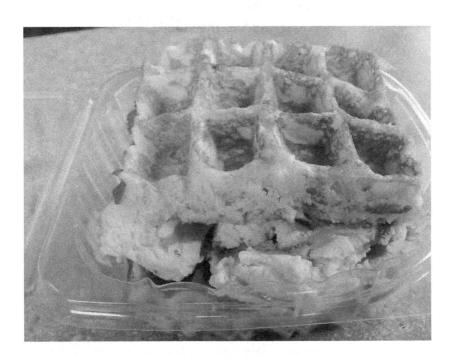

18. Tuna Sandwich Chaffles

Preparation time: 6 minutes

Cooking Time: 8 Minutes

Servings: 2

- **Ingredients:**
- Chaffles
- 1 organic egg, beaten
- ½ cup cheddar cheese, shredded
- 1 tablespoon almond flour
- Pinch of salt
- Filling
- ¼ cup water-packed tuna, flaked
- 2 lettuce leaves

Directions:

1. Preheat a mini waffle iron and then grease it.
2. For chaffles: In a medium bowl, put all ingredients and with a fork, mix until well combined. Place half of the mixture into preheated waffle iron and cook for about 3–4 minutes.
3. Repeat with the remaining mixture.
4. Serve each chaffle with filling ingredients.

Nutrition:

- Calories: 211
- Fat: 16 g
- Protein: 8 g
- Sugar: 0 g

19. Beef Chaffle Sandwich Recipe

Preparation time: 10 minutes

Cooking Time: 15 Minutes

Servings: 2

Ingredients:

- Batter
- 3 eggs
- 2 cups grated mozzarella cheese
- ¼ cup cream cheese
- Salt and pepper to taste
- 1 teaspoon Italian seasoning
- Beef
- 2 tablespoons butter
- 1 pound beef tenderloin
- Salt and pepper to taste
- 2 teaspoons Dijon mustard
- 1 teaspoon dried paprika
- Other
- 2 tablespoons cooking spray to brush the waffle maker
- 4 lettuce leaves for serving
- 4 tomato slices for serving
- 4 leaves fresh basil

Directions:

1. Preheat the waffle maker.
2. Add the eggs, grated mozzarella cheese, salt and pepper and Italian seasoning to a bowl.
3. Mix until combined and batter forms.

4. Brush the heated waffle maker with cooking spray and add a few tablespoons of the batter.
5. Close the lid and cook for about 7 minutes depending on your waffle maker.
6. Meanwhile, melt and heat the butter in a nonstick frying pan.
7. Season the beef loin with salt and pepper, brush it with Dijon mustard, and sprinkle some dried paprika on top.
8. Cook the beef on each side for about 5 minutes.
9. Thinly slice the beef and assemble the chaffle sandwiches.
10. Cut each chaffle in half and on one half place a lettuce leaf, tomato slice, basil leaf, and some sliced beef.
11. Cover with the other chaffle half and serve.

Nutrition:

- Calories: 96
- Fat: 6 g
- Protein: 4 g
- Sugar: 0 g

20. Sloppy Joe Chaffles

Preparation Time: 10 minutes

Cooking Time: 5 minutes

Servings: 4

Ingredients

- Sloppy jaw ingredients
- 1 lb. ground beef
- 1 tsp. onion powder
- 1 teaspoon of garlic
- 3 tbsp. tomato paste
- 1/2 teaspoon
- 1/4 teaspoon pepper
- Chili powder 1 tbs
- 1 teaspoon of cocoa powder this is optional but highly recommended! It enhances the flavor!
- Usually, 1/2 cup bone soup beef flavor
- 1 teaspoon coconut amino or soy sauce as you like
- 1 teaspoon mustard powder
- 1 teaspoon of brown or screen golden
- 1/2 teaspoon paprika
- Ingredients for corn bread chaffle
- 1 egg
- 1/2 cup cheddar cheese
- 5-slice jalapeno, very small diced (pickled or fresh)
- 1 tsp. frank red hot sauce
- 1/4 teaspoon corn extract is optional, but tastes like real cornbread!
- Pinch salt

Directions

1. First, cooking the minced meat with salt and pepper.
2. Add all remaining ingredients.
3. Cooking the mixture while making the chaffle.
4. Preheating waffle maker.
5. Put the eggs in a small bowl.
6. Add the remaining ingredients.
7. Spray to the waffle maker with a non-stick cooking spray.
8. Divide the mixture in half.
9. Simmer half of the mixture for about 4 minutes or until golden.
10. For a chaffle crispy rind, add 1 teaspoon cheese to the waffle maker for 30 seconds before adding the mixture.
11. Pour the warm stubby joe mix into the hot chaffle and finish! Dinner is ready!
12. Note: You can also add diced jalapenos (fresh or pickled) to this basic chaffle recipe to make a jalapeno cornbread chaffle recipe!

Nutrition:

- Calories: 96
- Fat: 1.3 g
- Protein: 7 g
- Sugar: 4.5 g

21. Pumpkin Cake Chaffle Plus Cream Cheese Frosting

Preparation Time: 15 minutes

Cooking Time: 28 minutes

Servings: 4

Ingredients

- For the pumpkin chaffles:
- 2 eggs, beaten
- ½ tsp. pumpkin pie spice
- 1 cup finely grated Mozzarella cheese
- 1 tbsp. pumpkin puree
- For the cream cheese frosting:
- 2 tbsp. cream cheese, softened
- 2 tbsp. swerve confectioner's sugar
- ½ tsp. vanilla extract

Directions

1. For the chaffles:
2. Preheat the waffle iron.
3. In a medium bowl, mix the egg, pumpkin pie spice, Mozzarella cheese, and pumpkin puree.
4. Open the iron and add a quarter of the mixture. Close and cooking until crispy, 7 minutes.
5. Transfer the chaffle to a plate and make 3 more chaffles with the remaining batter.
6. For the cream cheese frosting:
7. Add the cream cheese, swerve sugar, and vanilla to a medium bowl and whisk using an electric mixer until smooth and fluffy.

8. Layer the chaffles one on another but with some frosting spread between the layers. Top with the bit of frosting.
9. Slice and serve.

Nutrition:

- Calories: 340
- Protein: 50 g
- Carbohydrates: 14 g
- Fats: 10 g

22. S'mores Chaffle

Preparation Time: 15 minutes

Cooking Time: 28 minutes

Servings: 4

Ingredients

- 2 eggs, beaten
- 1 cup finely grated gruyere cheese
- ½ tsp. vanilla extract
- 2 tbsp. swerve brown sugar
- A pinch of salt
- ¼ cup unsweetened chocolate chips, melted
- 2 tbsp. low carb marshmallow fluff

Directions

1. Preheat the waffle iron.
2. In a medium bowl, mix the eggs, gruyere cheese, vanilla, swerve sugar, and salt.
3. Open the iron and add a quarter of the mixture. Close and cooking until crispy, 7 minutes.
4. Transfer the chaffle to a plate and make 3 more chaffles with the remaining batter.
5. Spread half of the chocolate on two chaffles, add the marshmallow fluff and cover with the other chaffles.
6. Swirl the remaining chocolate, slice in half and serve.

Nutrition:

- Calories: 303
- Protein: 15 g
- Carbohydrates: 30 g
- Fats: 14 g

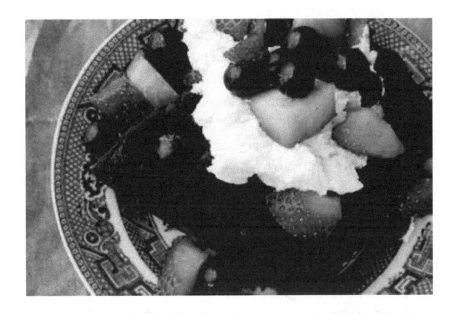

23. Chocolate Cake Chaffles Plus Cream Cheese Frosting

Preparation Time: 10 minutes

Cooking Time: 28 minutes

Servings: 4

Ingredients

- For the chaffles:
- 2 eggs, beaten
- 1 cup finely grated gouda cheese
- 2 tsp. unsweetened cocoa powder
- ¼ tsp. sugar-free maple syrup
- 1 tbsp. cream cheese, softened
- For the frosting:
- 3 tbsp. cream cheese, softened
- ¼ tsp. vanilla extract
- 2 tbsp. sugar-free maple syrup

Directions

1. For the chaffles:
2. Preheat the waffle iron.
3. In a medium bowl, mix all the ingredients for the chaffles.
4. Open the iron and add a quarter of the mixture. Close and cooking until crispy, 7 minutes.
5. Transfer the chaffle to a plate and make 3 more chaffles with the remaining batter.
6. For the frosting:

7. In a medium bowl, beat the cream cheese, vanilla extract, and maple syrup with a hand mixer until smooth.
8. Assemble the chaffles with the frosting to make the cake making sure to top the last layer with some frosting.
9. Slice and serve.

Nutrition:

- Calories: 350
- Protein: 51 g
- Carbohydrates: 10 g
- Fats: 10 g

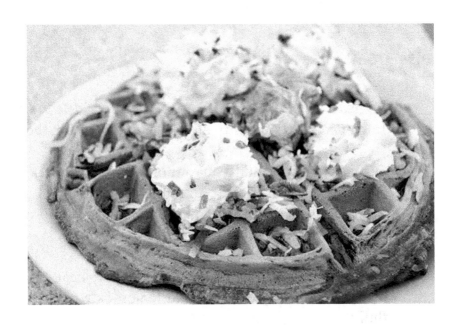

24. Lemon Cake Chaffle With Frosting

Preparation Time: 10 minutes

Cooking Time: 28 minutes

Servings: 4

Ingredients

- For the chaffles:
- 2 eggs, beaten
- ½ cup finely grated swiss cheese
- 2 oz. cream cheese, softened
- ½ tsp. lemon extract
- 20 drops cake batter extract
- For the frosting:
- ½ cup heavy cream
- 1 tbsp. sugar-free maple syrup
- ¼ tsp. lemon extract

Directions

1. For the chaffles:
2. Preheat the waffle iron.
3. In a medium bowl, mix all the ingredients for the chaffles.
4. Open the iron and add a quarter of the mixture. Close and cooking until crispy, 7 minutes.
5. Transfer the chaffle to a plate and make 3 more chaffles with the remaining batter.
6. For the frosting:
7. In a medium bowl, using a hand mixer, beat the heavy cream, maple syrup, and lemon extract until fluffy.

8. Assemble the chaffles with the frosting to make the cake.
9. Slice and serve.

Nutrition:

- Calories: 149
- Protein: 17 g
- Carbohydrates: 4.5 g
- Fats: 6 g

SAVORY CHAFFLE RECIPES

25. Spicy Black Sesame Chaffles

Preparation Time: 10 minutes

Cooking Time: 10 minutes

Servings: 4

Ingredients:

- 2 cups almond flour
- 2 cups almond milk
- Juice of ½ lemon
- 1/3 cup black sesame seeds
- A pinch of salt and black pepper
- 2 eggs, whisked
- 1 teaspoon chili powder
- 1 teaspoon hot paprika

Directions:

1. In a bowl mix the almond flour with the almond milk and the other ingredients and whisk well.
2. Heat up the waffle iron, pour ¼ of the batter and cooking for 10 minutes.
3. Repeat with the rest of the mix and serve.

Nutrition:

- Calories: 69
- Fat: 4.9 g
- Fiber: 2.1 g
- Carbs: 5.4 g
- Protein: 2.4 g

26.   Spicy Zucchini Chaffles

Preparation Time: 10 minutes

Cooking Time: 8 minutes

Servings: 6

Ingredients:

- 1 and ½ cups almond flour
- 2 teaspoons baking powder
- 2 eggs, whisked
- 1 and ½ cups coconut milk
- 2 zucchinis, grated
- 1 teaspoon chili powder
- 1 teaspoon cayenne pepper
- 1 cup cheddar cheese, shredded

Directions:

1. In a bowl, mix the almond flour with the eggs, milk and the other ingredients and whisk well.
2. Preheat the waffle iron, pour 1/6 of the batter, cooking the chaffle for 8 minutes and transfer to a plate.
3. Repeat with the rest of the batter and serve.

Nutrition:

- Calories: 50
- Fat: 2.9 g
- Fiber: 6.6 g
- Carbs: 0.1 g
- Protein: 0.7 g

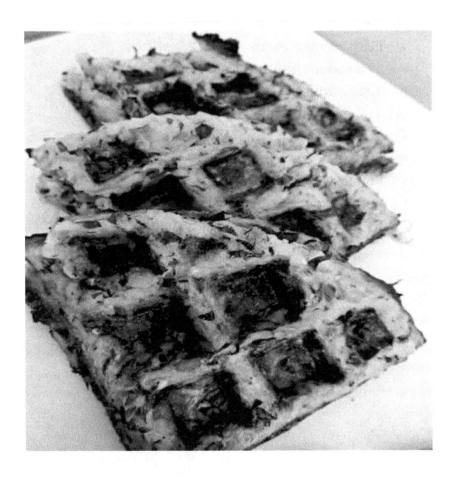

27. Tabasco Chaffle

Preparation Time: 5 minutes

Cooking Time: 8 minutes

Servings: 4

Ingredients:

- 1 cup coconut milk
- 1 cup coconut flour
- 2 teaspoons Tabasco sauce
- 2 eggs, whisked
- 2 tablespoons ghee, melted
- ½ cup mozzarella, shredded
- 1 teaspoon cayenne pepper
- 1 tablespoon chives, chopped
- 1 tablespoon baking powder
- A pinch of salt and black pepper

Directions:

1. In a bowl, mix the milk with the flour, Tabasco sauce and the other ingredients and whisk well.
2. Preheat the waffle iron, pour ¼ of the batter, cooking for 8 minutes and transfer to a plate.
3. Repeat with the rest of the batter and serve.

Nutrition:

- Calories: 71
- Fat: 1.9 g
- Fiber: 5.9 g
- Carbs: 13 g
- Protein: 3g

28. Green Cayenne Chaffle

Preparation Time: 10 minutes

Cooking Time: 10 minutes

Servings: 4

Ingredients:

- 1 cup coconut flour
- ½ cup cream cheese, soft
- ½ cup coconut milk
- 1 tablespoon chives, chopped
- 1 tablespoon parsley, chopped
- 1 green chili pepper, minced
- ½ teaspoon cayenne pepper
- 1 teaspoon baking soda

Directions:

1. In a bowl, mi the eggs with the cream cheese, milk and the other ingredients and whisk well.
2. Preheat the waffle iron, pour ¼ of the batter, close the waffle maker, cooking for 10 minutes and transfer to a plate.
3. Repeat with the rest of the batter and serve.

Nutrition:

- Calories: 44
- Fat: 3 g
- Fiber: 1.8 g
- Carbs: 4.3 g
- Protein: 1 g

29. Hot Pesto Chaffles

Preparation Time: 10 minutes

Cooking Time: 7 minutes

Servings: 4

Ingredients:

- 1 cup almond milk
- 1 cup mozzarella, shredded
- 1 cup coconut flour
- 3 tablespoons basil pesto
- 1 teaspoon hot paprika
- 1 teaspoon chili powder
- 2 eggs, whisked
- 1 tablespoon ghee, melted
- 1 teaspoon baking soda

Directions:

1. In a bowl, mix the milk with the cheese, pesto and the other ingredients and whisk.
2. Heat up the waffle maker, pour ¼ of the mix, cooking for 7 minutes and transfer to a plate.
3. Repeat with the rest of the mix and serve.

Nutrition:

- Calories: 101
- Fat: 7.4 g
- Fiber: 3.2 g
- Carbs: 8.3 g
- Protein: 3.1g

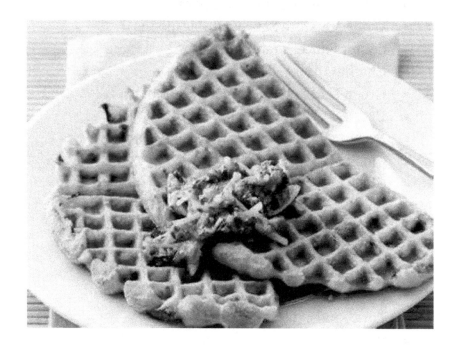

30. Katsu Chaffle Sandwich

Preparation time: 90 minutes

Cooking Time: 22 minutes

Servings: 2

Ingredients:

- Sauce
- Ketchup: 2 tablespoons (sugar-free)
- Swerve/Monk fruit: 1 teaspoon
- Worcestershire Sauce: 2 tablespoons
- Oyster Sauce: 1 tablespoon
- Chaffle
- Green Leaf Lettuce: 2 leaves (optional)
- Egg: 2
- Mozzarella cheese: 1 cup (shredded)
- Chicken
- Chicken thigh: 2 pieces boneless or ¼ lb. boneless
- Egg: 1
- Black pepper: ¼ teaspoon or as per your taste
- Vegetable oil: 2 cups (deep frying)
- Almond flour: 1 cup
- Salt: ¼ teaspoon or as per your taste
- Pork Rinds: 3 oz. unflavored
- Brine
- Water: 2 cups
- Salt: 1 tablespoon

Directions:

1. Using a skillet, boil the chicken with salt and 2 cups of water.
2. With the lid closed, boil for 28 minutes.

3. Once done, dry the chicken using a small towel to pat, then add salt and dried pepper on its sides.
4. Using a mixing bowl, a mixture containing the oyster sauce, monk fruit, sugar-free ketchup and Worcestershire and set aside.
5. Using a food processor or blender, grind the pork rinds to fine crumbs.
6. Using 3 mixing bowls containing the ingredients respectively (Almond flour, beaten eggs in another and the crushed pork in the last), coat the chicken using the ingredients in these bowls in this order (Flour-Eggs-Pork).
7. Deep fry the chicken pieces in a frying pan to a golden brown, then place in a rack for excess oil to drip out.
8. Using another mixing bowl, a mix containing shredded Mozzarella cheese with beaten eggs. With a closed lid, mix evenly and heat the waffle for 5 minutes to a crunch.
9. Once timed out, remove the chaffle from the waffle maker.
10. Repeat for the remaining chaffles mixture.
11. Slice the avocados with the green leaf lettuce washed and dried.
12. With one chaffle, spread sauce on it, the green lettuce, chicken katsu and close with another chaffle. Serve the dish and savor the taste.

Nutrition:

- Calories: 187
- Fat: 14.8 g
- Carbs: 4.7 g
- Protein: 9.5 g

31. **Bread Sandwich Chaffle**

Preparation time: 18 minutes

Cooking Time: 12 minutes

Servings: 2

Ingredients:

- Almond flour: 1 tablespoon
- Mayo: 2 tablespoons
- Garlic powder: ½ teaspoon
- Egg: 2
- Water: 2 teaspoons
- Baking powder: 1/8 teaspoon

Directions:

1. a mix of ingredients in a mixing bowl. Preheat and grease the waffle maker.
2. Pour in the mixture into the waffle maker and spread evenly.
3. Heat the mixture to a crispy form.
4. Repeat the process to make as many chaffles as possible from the remaining.

Nutrition:

- Calories: 61
- Fat: 2.6 g
- Fiber: 3.2 g
- Carbs: 8.1 g
- Protein: 3.4 g

32. Chaffle Sandwich With Eggs and Bacon

Preparation time: 12 minutes

Cooking Time: 6 minutes

Servings: 2

Ingredients:

- Sandwich
- Bacon strips: 4
- Egg: 2
- American cheese: 2 slices
- Chaffles
- Egg: 2
- Cheddar cheese: 1 cup (shredded)

Directions:

1. Preheat and grease the waffle maker.
2. Using a mixing bowl, a mix containing shredded cheddar with beaten eggs.
3. Blend to a froth, then add the earlier chocolate mixture.
4. Mix evenly and pour into the lower side of the waffle maker.
5. With a closed lid, heat the waffle for 5 minutes to a crunch and then remove the chaffle.
6. Heat the sliced bacon to a crispy form using medium heat in a non-stick large pan, drain the fried bacon then fry the eggs.
7. Put off the heat on the chaffle. Repeat for the remaining chaffles mixture to make more batter.

8. Serve egg and cheese with slices of bacon in between two chaffles and enjoy.

Nutrition:

- Calories: 48
- Fat: 2.5 g
- Fiber: 2.6 g
- Carbs: 5.7 g
- Protein: 1.9 g

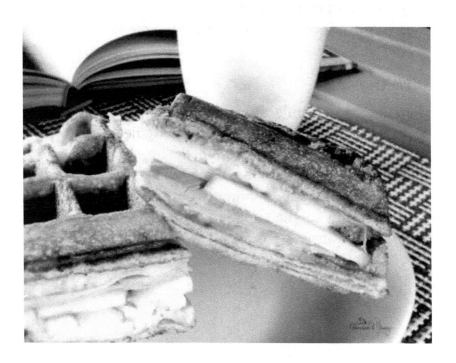

SPECIAL CHAFFLE RECIPES

33. Protein Mozzarella Chaffles

Preparation time: 8 minutes

Cooking Time: 20 Minutes

Servings: 2

Ingredients:

- ½ scoop unsweetened protein powder
- 2 large organic eggs
- ½ cup Mozzarella cheese, shredded
- 1 tablespoon Erythritol
- ¼ teaspoon organic vanilla extract

Directions:

1. Preheat a mini waffle iron and then grease it.
2. In a medium bowl, place all ingredients and with a fork, mix until well combined.
3. Place ¼ of the mixture into preheated waffle iron and cook for about 4-5 minutes or until golden brown.
4. Repeat with the remaining mixture.
5. Serve warm.

Nutrition:

- Calories: 400
- Fat: 21 g
- Cholesterol: 0 mg
- Carbohydrates: 46 g
- Sugar: 2 g
- Fiber: 3 g
- Protein: 11 g
- Sodium: 6 mg
- Calcium: 64 mg
- Phosphorus: 113 mg
- Potassium: 202 mg

34. Chocolate Chips Peanut Butter Chaffles

Preparation time: 5 minutes

Cooking Time: 8 Minutes

Servings: 4

Ingredients:

- 1 organic egg, beaten
- ¼ cup Mozzarella cheese, shredded
- 2 tablespoons creamy peanut butter
- 1 tablespoon almond flour
- 1 tablespoon granulated Erythritol
- 1 teaspoon organic vanilla extract
- 1 tablespoon 70% dark chocolate chips

Directions:

1. Preheat a mini waffle iron and then grease it.
2. In a bowl, place all ingredients except chocolate chips and beat until well combined.
3. Gently, fold in the chocolate chips.
4. Place half of the mixture into preheated waffle iron and cook for about minutes or until golden brown.
5. Repeat with the remaining mixture.
6. Serve warm.

Nutrition:

- Calories 47
- Fat: 1 g
- Cholesterol: 0 g
- Carbohydrates: 8 g
- Sugar: 6 g
- Fiber: 2 g
- Protein 2 g
- Sodium: 104 mg
- Calcium: 36 mg
- Phosphorus: 52 mg
- Potassium: 298 mg

35. <u>Dessert Pumpkin Chaffles</u>

Preparation time: 5 minutes

Cooking Time: 12 Minutes

Servings: 3

Ingredients:

- 1 organic egg, beaten
- ½ cup Mozzarella cheese, shredded
- 1½ tablespoon homemade pumpkin puree
- ½ teaspoon Erythritol
- ½ teaspoon organic vanilla extract
- ¼ teaspoon pumpkin pie spice

Directions:

1. Preheat a mini waffle iron and then grease it.
2. In a bowl, place all the ingredients and beat until well combined.
3. Place ¼ of the mixture into preheated waffle iron and cook for about 4-6 minutes or until golden brown.
4. Repeat with the remaining mixture.
5. Serve warm.

Nutrition:

- Calories: 300
- Fat: 19 g
- Cholesterol: 0 mg
- Carbohydrates: 34 g
- Sugar: 11 g
- Fiber: 5 g
- Protein: 6 g
- Sodium: 6 mg
- Calcium: 30 mg
- Phosphorus: 144 mg
- Potassium: 296 mg

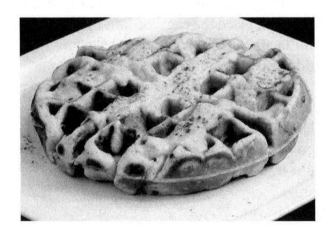

36. Chocolate Chips Chaffles

Preparation time: 5 minutes

Cooking Time: 8 Minutes

Servings: 2

Ingredients:

- 1 large organic egg
- 1 teaspoon coconut flour
- 1 teaspoon Erythritol
- ½ teaspoon organic vanilla extract
- ½ cup Mozzarella cheese, shredded finely
- 2 tablespoons 70% dark chocolate chips

Directions:

1. Preheat a mini waffle iron and then grease it.
2. In a bowl, place the egg, coconut flour, sweetener and vanilla extract and beat until well combined.
3. Add the cheese and stir to combine.
4. Place half of the mixture into preheated waffle iron and top with half of the chocolate chips.
5. Place a little egg mixture over each chocolate chip.
6. Cook for about 3-4 minutes or until golden brown.
7. Repeat with the remaining mixture and chocolate chips.
8. Serve warm.

Nutrition:

- Calories: 156
- Fat: 12 g
- Cholesterol: 42 mg
- Carbohydrates: 4 g
- Sugar: 2 g
- Fiber: 0 g
- Protein: 14 g
- Sodium: 48 mg
- Calcium: 18 mg
- Phosphorus: 114 mg
- Potassium: 220 mg

37. Cream Cake Chaffles

Preparation time: 8 minutes

Cooking Time: 12 Minutes

Servings: 2

Ingredients:

- Chaffle
- 4 oz cream cheese, softened
- 4 eggs
- 4 tbsp coconut flour
- 1 tbsp almond flour
- 1 ½ tsp baking powder
- 1 tbsp butter, softened
- 1 tsp vanilla extract
- ½ tsp cinnamon
- 1 tbsp sweetener
- 1 tbsp shredded coconut, colored and unsweetened
- 1 tbsp walnuts, chopped
- Italian Cream Frosting
- 2 oz cream cheese, softened
- 2 tbsp butter, room temperature
- 2 tbsp sweetener
- ½ tsp vanilla

Directions:

1. Preheat your waffle maker and add ¼ of the
2. Cook for 3 minutes and repeat the process until you have 4 chaffles.
3. Remove and set aside.

4. In the meantime, start making your frosting by mixing all the
5. Stir until you have a smooth and creamy mixture.
6. Cool, frost the cake and enjoy.

Nutrition:
- Calories: 149
- Fat: 8 g
- Cholesterol: 0 mg
- Carbohydrates: 18 g
- Sugar: 15 g
- Fiber: 4 g
- Protein: 3 g
- Sodium: 76 mg
- Calcium: 73 mg
- Phosphorus: 26 mg

38. Almond & Butter Chaffles

Preparation time: 5 minutes

Cooking Time: 10 Minutes

Servings: 2

Ingredients:

- 1 large organic egg, beaten
- 1/3 cup Mozzarella cheese, shredded
- 1 tablespoon Erythritol
- 2 tablespoons almond butter
- 1 teaspoon organic vanilla extract

Directions:

1. Preheat a mini waffle iron and then grease it.
2. In a medium bowl, place all ingredients and with a fork, mix until well combined.
3. Place half of the mixture into preheated waffle iron and cook for about 5 minutes or until golden brown.
4. Repeat with the remaining mixture.
5. Serve warm.

Nutrition:

- Calories: 365
- Fat: 11 g
- Cholesterol: 0 mg
- Carbohydrate: 58 g
- Sugar: 11 g
- Fiber: 4 g
- Protein: 9 g
- Sodium: 95 mg
- Calcium: 41 mg
- Phosphorus: 119 mg
- Potassium: 264 mg

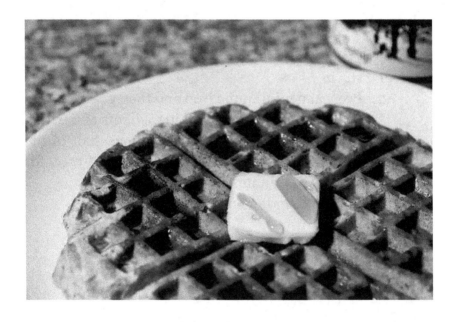

39. Simple Mozzarella Chaffles

Preparation time: 5 minutes

Cooking Time: 8 Minutes

Servings: 2

Ingredients:

- ½ cup mozzarella cheese, shredded
- 1 large organic egg
- 2 tablespoons blanched almond flour
- ¼ teaspoon organic baking powder
- 2–3 drops liquid

Directions:

1. stevia
2. Preheat a mini waffle iron and then grease it.
3. In a medium bowl, put all ingredients and with a fork, mix until well combined. Place half of the mixture into preheated waffle iron and cook for about 3–4 minutes.
4. Repeat with the remaining mixture.
5. Serve warm.

Nutrition:

- Calories: 61
- Fat: 2 g
- Carb: 9 g
- Phosphorus: 23 mg
- Potassium: 178 mg
- Sodium: 98 mg
- Protein: 2 g

40. Cream Mini-Chaffles

Preparation time: 5 minutes

Cooking Time: 10 Minutes

Servings: 2

Ingredients:

- 2 tsp coconut flour
- 4 tsp swerve/monk fruit
- ¼ tsp baking powder
- 1 egg
- 1 oz cream cheese
- ½ tsp vanilla extract

Directions:

1. Turn on waffle maker to heat and oil it with cooking spray.
2. Mix swerve/monk fruit, coconut flour, and baking powder in a small mixing bowl.
3. Add cream cheese, egg, vanilla extract, and whisk until well-combined.
4. Add batter into waffle maker and cook for 3-minutes, until golden brown.
5. Serve with your favorite toppings.

Nutrition:

- Calories: 51
- Fat: 2 g
- Carb: 9 g
- Phosphorus: 63 mg
- Potassium: 198 mg
- Sodium: 128 mg
- Protein: 2 g

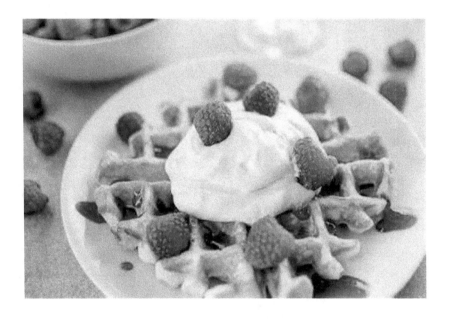

CONCLUSION

Chaffles is the amazing new invention you've been waiting for. It's a revolutionary, patent-pending, and 100% vegan protein bar with a thousand uses.

What are chaffles? Chaffles is a delicious new product that can be used to replace the high fat and high sugar snacks in your diet like cheese chips or chocolate bars. It's also gluten-free, vegan, non-GMO, low in sodium and preservative free! The best part is that chaffles taste just as good as candy! You'll never want anything else again after trying this life changing snack.

The combination of protein and savory chaffle taste will keep you wanting to eat more every time. Chaffles are also a great substitute for those times that you feel like having something sweet, but want something healthy with a lot of flavor.

Chaffles come in an assortment of flavors like Pecan Pie or Cherry Pie and can be served with a drizzle of your favorite nut butter or cinnamon sugar for an awesome snack. Or you can create your own combinations by mixing them up the way that makes your mouth water.

Chaffles are great for both kids and adults. They're the perfect snack to bring on a hike for an afternoon treat or to eat on a road trip or flights. Even better, they create a new way for parents to get their kids to eat protein without them even knowing what they're eating. Now if you want your children to enjoy healthy food without complaining, chaffles will be your best friend.

No matter what you eat chaffles with, it will never disappoint! Have it with chicken noodle soup or mashed potatoes for dinner or have it with salad at lunch.

Chaffle is a perfect combination for keto dieters. Besides, keto diet is always low in carbs and high in fat so chaffle is an amazing option for it.

Chaffles are very versatile and can be used as a spread for your favorite bagel or toast, or even on top of a pizza before baking it. You can also use chaffles as an ingredient for your own meals like pancakes, pies, donuts, breads and so much more!

Chaffle comes in two different flavors: savory and sweet. The savory flavor is more of a BBQ flavor while the sweet flavor is more cookie dough style. The savory chaffles are perfect for replacing things like bread and crackers, while sweet chaffles can be used as a dessert or drink! You can also add chaffle to your favorite dessert recipes for an amazing taste.

Chaffles are the most unique tasting protein bar around that is also good for you. You won't believe how good they taste until you try them for yourself. This incredible product is sure to revolutionize your snacking experience and change the way you think about eating healthy forever.

Always remember when making your own chaffle recipes, you can choose from almost any combination of things like fruits, cereals, nuts and seeds. You can even use different types of chocolate in some recipes. Anything goes with chaffle!

What's even more exciting is that chaffles come in many sizes to fit anyone's taste and diet.

It's time to ditch your unhealthy snacks for life changing chaffles!

CPSIA information can be obtained
at www.ICGtesting.com
Printed in the USA
BVHW092323240621
610373BV00004B/1134

9 781802 349009